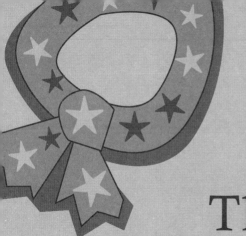

The
Ultimate
SCARF
Book

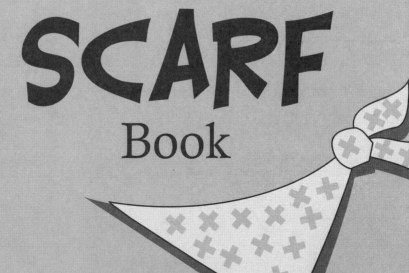

RUNNING PRESS
PHILADELPHIA · LONDON

ISBN 0-7624-1465-0

Package, book cover, interior design, and illustrations by Corinda Cook
Package photography by Steve Mullen
Text by Conn McQuinn
Edited by Elizabeth Shiflett
Typography: Calisto, Jacoby, and Mod

Package flap and p. 29: Sunflowers, painting by Vincent van Gogh. Neue Pinakothek, Munich, Germany;
Scala/Art Resource, NY.

This kit containing this book may be ordered by mail from the publisher.
Please include $2.50 for postage and handling.
But try your bookstore first!

Running Press Book Publishers
125 South Twenty-second Street
Philadelphia, Pennsylvania 19103-4399

Visit us on the web!
www.runningpress.com

CONTENTS

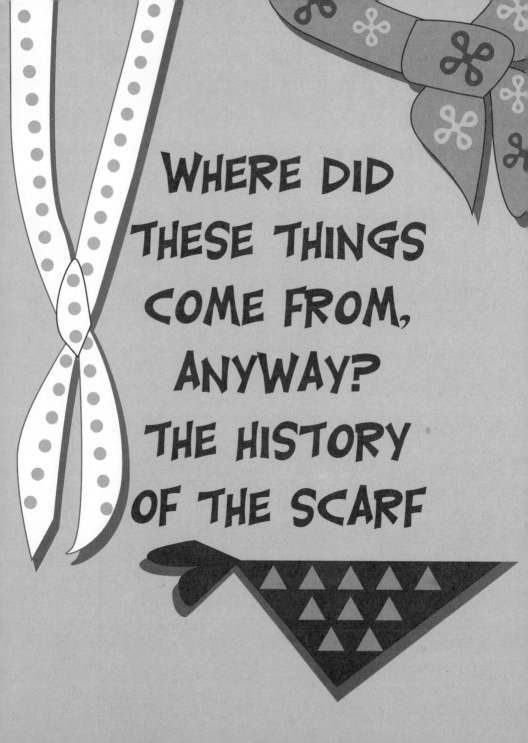

WHERE DID THESE THINGS COME FROM, ANYWAY? THE HISTORY OF THE SCARF

Scarves have been around for thousands of years. In fact, a basic scarf was probably among the first types of clothing used by man. A scarf is just a square piece of fabric, after all! One of the oldest garments ever recovered was a large scarf woven from horsehair that was found in an Irish bog. Tests indicated that it was over 5,000 years old!

Images and sculptures from many ancient civilizations show women (and men) wearing scarf-like fashions on their heads or around their necks. However, the scarf as we know it today didn't really become possible until the discovery of silk.

Silk is made from the cocoons of a caterpillar. According to legend, it was accidentally discovered in 2460 B.C. by the bride of the Chinese emperor, Princess His-ling-shi. One day a cocoon dropped into her tea (or into her bathtub, in some versions of the story). When she went to pull it out, the cocoon began to unravel into a fine thread. This thread was then woven into a new kind of fabric that was thin, light, and incredibly smooth to the touch. The new material could be dyed with many bright colors.

Soon, this miracle fabric was traded all around the world. Silk became so valuable that how it was made was considered a government secret. For over 2,000 years China was the only country that produced silk. Eventually, however, merchants were able to smuggle silkworms to Japan

YEE HAW!

and India. In A.D. 552, two monks visiting China hid eggs in their walking sticks and carried them all the way back to Europe for Emperor Justinian. From there, silk production spread to any country where the silkworms could survive.

Scarves that we would recognize today began to appear in European paintings as early as the 1600s. They were often colorful additions to hats, either used as decoration or tied to keep the hat from falling off. During that time, men also wore fancy scarves, called cravats, around their necks. This early version of the necktie was part of many military uniforms.

Over the years, scarves have been used as head coverings, wrapped around the neck for warmth, draped across the shoulders like a shawl, or just added for decoration. In the American west, cowboys and outlaws even used a scarf-like cloth called a bandanna to keep dust out of their faces—or to hide their faces during a holdup! Fashions have come and gone, but the basic scarf always seems to find a way to stay popular.

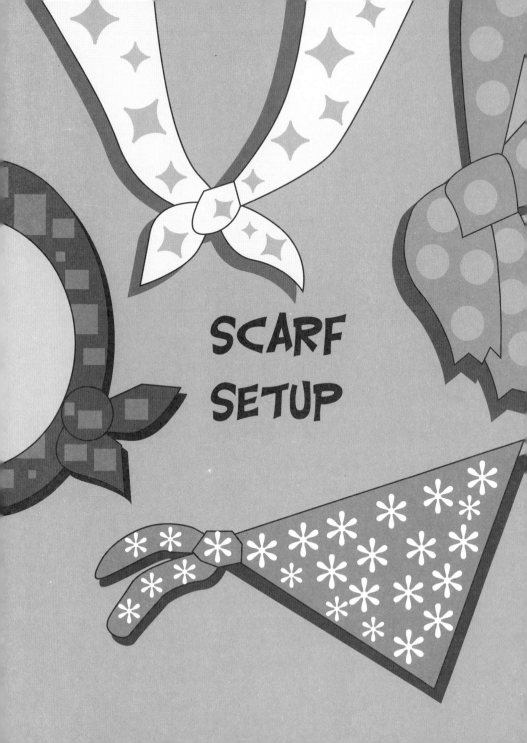

SCARF SETUP

Getting Ready

Painting can be a lot of fun, but it can also be a big mess. Make sure you set up your space for working by doing these things:

✳ Put a plastic garbage bag on your work surface and lay some newspapers on top in case you spill.

✳ Have rags or paper towels ready.

✳ Wear old clothes that don't matter if they get stained.

✳ Keep the plastic mixing tray from this kit handy for mixing your paints, or use plastic plates. The plastic surface won't absorb the paint.

✳ Use an old cereal bowl of water for rinsing out your brush. (Bowls are harder to accidentally tip over than cups are.)

Careful setup will help make sure that the scarf gets painted, instead of the dining room table or the carpet!

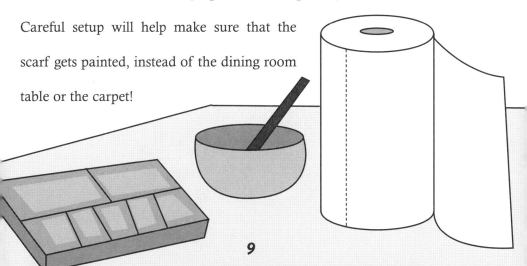

Practice, Practice, Practice

Your kit comes with two practice paper sheets, one for each scarf. Use these practice sheets to experiment with different designs or techniques. (You can photocopy or trace the scarf outlines to make more than one practice run.) Practice drawing your designs on the paper scarves with crayons or markers and save the special paint for a small test sheet and the actual scarves. You only have two scarves to decorate, so you want to make sure you have a good idea of what to paint before starting on the real fabric. Practicing on the paper will also allow you to make mistakes where it won't matter. Then you can have your best work on the scarf itself.

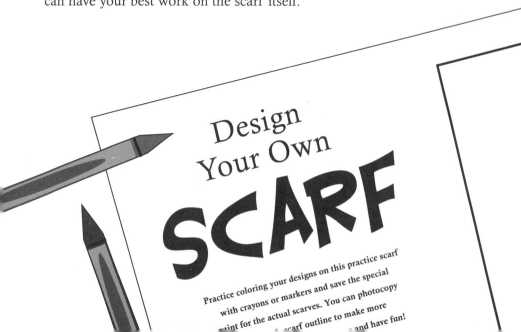

Design
Your Own
SCARF

Practice coloring your designs on this practice scarf with crayons or markers and save the special paint for the actual scarves. You can photocopy ....int for the actual scarves. You can photocopy ... scarf outline to make more ... and have fun!

Practice is important because these fabric paints are probably a bit different from other paints you may have used. These paints are made to be very watery so they will spread out on the fabric (and on your practice paper). Don't worry if the scarves don't come out exactly as you planned. Many scarf decorators try to make the paint spread even more to make cool patterns on the fabric! Be creative and have fun. Not matter what you do, it will be a one-of-a-kind masterpiece made especially by you!

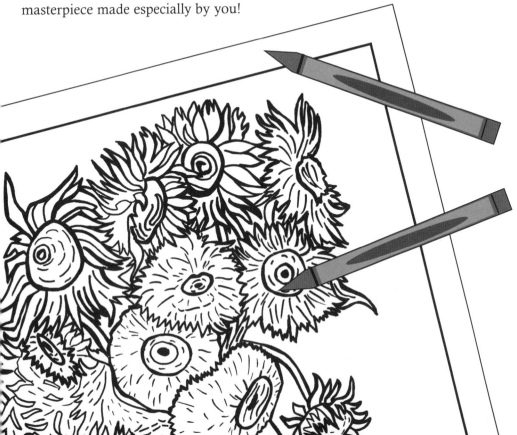

Designing Your Scarves

Scarves can have almost any kind of design. Some have a picture painted on them, while others are decorated with abstract patterns of color or even a few lines that make a symbol or drawing. In your kit, you have two scarves. The smaller, square one has a famous painting on it for you to color, while the longer, rectangular one is ready for your own original design.

You might want to start with the pre-printed scarf to practice using the paints. Or you can also make a perfectly beautiful design of your own on the blank scarf using some of the techniques in this book. Before you start either scarf, you'll probably want to think about what colors, design, and techniques you want to use.

If you have a chance, the next time you're at the mall, drop in to a store that sells scarves. Take a look at some of the different ideas that the professional designers have come up with and see what looks good to you. (There will be lots of choices if you look before Christmas or Mother's Day!) You'll notice that some scarves have detailed pictures on them, but others are dyed in random colors that all blend together into a lovely design. Use these scarves for inspiration, but don't be limited by what you see. Be creative!

Think about the person you're making the scarf for, and what kind of scarf you'd like to make for them. You may find it helpful to brainstorm ideas for your scarves before trying to draw the design. When you brainstorm, you think of as many ideas as you can and write them down on a piece of paper. No idea is a bad one at this stage—even one that seems silly at first could inspire you to think of one that might work better. What does the special person you're making the scarf for like? What colors does she like? What are her hobbies? What kind of job does she have? Does she have a favorite animal or pet? Does she love nature, trees, or flowers? After you've made your list, read it again and pick out the ideas you like best. As you design the scarf, you can try to think of ways to reflect her interests in the images that you create.

When you're creating a design, you should also decide whether you want to make one big picture that will cover the entire scarf, or divide it into parts. Many scarves have smaller pictures in different sections that all reflect an overall theme. You could choose several ideas from your brainstorming list and paint them onto different parts of the scarf for a special gift. When you're thinking about the scarf design, also decide whether or not you want to paint a border around the outside of the scarf, or even around each smaller picture you draw.

Keep in mind that these fabric paints are meant to bleed, or spread, on the fabric, so don't worry if your drawing doesn't turn out exactly the way you thought it would. The soft edges of the painted lines will actually help hide any mistakes you might make, so relax and have fun! The colors will also blend together when they touch each other, so you might want to leave some empty white space between two colors if you don't want them to mix together. You can even use the white space as a border or outline!

Whatever technique you use, mistakes will happen. Unlike some other surfaces, the scarf material soaks up the paint immediately, so you can't "erase" paint that does the wrong thing. Don't try to cover up your mistake with a lot of dark colors, as too many colors will look muddy brown. If you use your imagination, you can probably turn your mistake into a working part of the painting. Many artists have found that a "mistake" can end up making their work of art more special.

Brushing Up Your Technique

Your kit came with two bamboo paintbrushes. Before you start to paint your scarves, it's a good idea to practice using these brushes on another surface. Bamboo brushes work well with the watery paints used for scarf painting. They are better at holding liquid than other brushes you may have used before.

A new, dry bamboo brush comes with the brush bristles stuck together into a point and covered by a protective top. When you get the brush wet, the brush bristles will separate and become fuller, looking more like a regular paintbrush. Once this happens, the brush will hold a lot of water or watery paint. Bamboo brushes are perfect for making smooth, even lines without hard edges. However, they are not as good for painting small details or thin outlines.

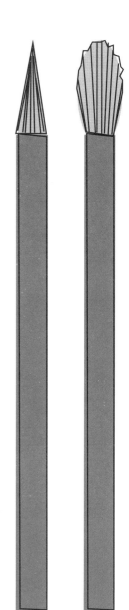

Bamboo Brush Dry   **Bamboo Brush Wet**

15

You're not limited to using the paintbrushes in the kit. If you have brushes of your own, you can paint with those, too. Different types of brushes can give different effects. Using a larger, flatter brush can save you time if you are painting large areas of the scarf with the same color. A flatter brush can also make the line you draw look different from a bamboo brush's line, because of the shape of the bristles and the amount of paint they hold. Some brushes that don't hold as much water may even add texture to your painting, because there may be areas where there is more paint than others. Sponge brushes are also good for painting large areas or making thick lines. They will give a different kind of line than a flat paintbrush because they hold more water and don't have bristles.

A very small, thin brush may make a more detailed line, but remember that these paints and the scarf material are meant to make the colors bleed, or spread out. If you're trying to make a thinner line, keep the brush as dry as you can. Only use a small amount of paint, and dab the brush lightly with a paper towel or newspaper if the brush looks too wet. Save the details until last, and wait until the scarf is completely dry to help minimize the bleeding.

Finally, don't be discouraged if the paint still spreads a bit!

You may want to practice using these different types of brushes before you use them on your special scarf! Trying them out on a piece of paper can help you choose which brush you want to use for different parts of your design. Practicing can also teach you many ways of using the same brush to get different results. Some of the projects described later don't use brushes at all. They may use folding, dipping, or other techniques. Even in the projects where you might normally use a brush, you can try another approach, such as sponging.

No matter which types of brushes you are using, make sure you rinse them out well when you switch colors of paint to prevent mixing. And don't mash the brushes down into the water to clean them out—they will last a long longer if you swish them instead. (I'm *sure* Leonardo da Vinci never mashed his brushes!)

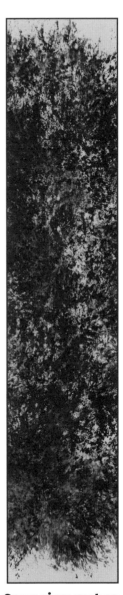

Sponging makes an unusual texture!

It's a Colorful World

Your kit comes with five colors—red, orange, yellow, green, and blue—and a mixing tray to hold the paint. This color choice may be perfect for the design you have in mind. But, if your imagination is calling for polka dots in a special shade of purple, you can try mixing the paints to get the color you want. By following a few hints about mixing colors, you'll have an endless choice of colors to use on your scarf!

Unless you're planning a scarf that's all one color, you'll probably want to start by putting a small amount of each color of paint into separate sections of the mixing tray or onto disposable plastic plates. Then, carefully put the lids back on the paint tubes so they don't spill. You won't have to worry about accidentally spilling all of your paint or dipping a dirty brush into your paint tube. While you're painting, if you need more of one color of paint, you can pour a little more into that section of the mixing tray.

When mixing colors, remember the color wheel. Red, yellow, and blue are the three primary colors. When red is mixed with yellow, you'll get orange. Yellow and blue makes green. Mixing red and blue can create purple. By care-

COLOR WHEEL

fully mixing small amounts of the paint colors together, you can experiment to see what colors you can create! But be careful not to mix too many colors together or the combined color will end up a muddy color of brown or black.

RED PURPLE

ORANGE BLUE

YELLOW GREEN

The best way to mix colors is by adding very small amounts of colors at a time, especially the darker ones. Remember that you can always add a little more color, but you can't take the paint you added back out of the mix.

If you just want a lighter version of a paint color, you can add drops of the paint to a small amount of clean water. For example, if you want to make a light pink color, dip a clean brush into the red section of your mixing tray. Then, swirl the brush in clean water in another section of your mixing tray. Keep adding more red and mixing until the pink color looks good to you. With patience and small amounts of paint, you can create almost any color you can imagine!

Get Ready, Get Set, But Before You Paint...

To properly paint your scarf, you'll need to set it up the right way. Make sure you work somewhere where spilling water or paint won't be a disaster. (For instance, the fancy dining room table is NOT a good place to do this!) Ask an adult to help you find the right place to get creative.

Your kit comes with small stretcher sponges that are sticky on both sides. The stretcher sponges are for holding your scarf above the surface of your work area. You will stick the stretcher sponges on the paper or plastic that covers your table or counter, then use the sticky topside to hold the corners of your scarf.

Lay your scarf out on the place where you will be painting. Slip the four stretcher sponges under the four corners of the scarf so that the edges of the stretcher sponges stick out just a little bit. Move the scarf, and then, one at a time, peel the backing from one side of each sponge and stick them down where you arranged them.

When all four stretcher sponges are secured to the work surface, stick the corners of the scarf onto the stretcher sponges. Keep the fabric tight, stretching it so it sits above the table and paper, and doesn't sag. If the scarf touches the paper or the table, it can cause the colors to run into each other, making a muddy color that's not even.

If you're planning to use a technique that involves folding or dipping your scarf into the paint, you may not want to put it on the stretcher sponges yet. After you finish painting the folded scarf or dipping it, allow the scarf to dry completely. Then, you can still stretch the scarf on the stretcher sponges if you'd like to use other decorating methods as well.

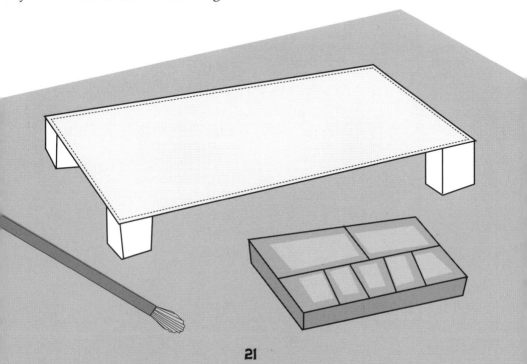

Wet or Dry?

When you paint on fabric with this type of paint, you can get different effects from the colors by leaving the fabric dry, or by wetting it down before you start. On a dry scarf, the lines you draw may stay more crisp and clean. That doesn't mean the paint will stay exactly where you touch the brush—it will probably still bleed a bit, but not too much. A wet scarf will make the colors spread much more freely, making fun patterns and very soft designs. The amount of water you use on the scarf will also affect the way the paint moves on the fabric.

To wet the scarf, you can use several different methods. Each one is good for certain painting techniques, and will make the paint spread in different ways. If you'd like the paint to spread very easily over the fabric, you can put the entire scarf into clean water. Then, squeeze out the extra water so the scarf doesn't drip too much. This method will make it more difficult to attach the scarf to the stretcher sponges. You might want to ask an adult to help you pin the edges of the scarf to the stretcher sponges. You can also just dip part of the scarf into the water if you only want the spreading effect in a certain area.

Another wetting method is using a sponge or brush to wet the cloth. First you should spread the scarf out on the stretcher sponges. Then, dip a sponge or a brush in clean water, gently shake off extra water, and "paint" the scarf with the water. This works well if you want to control where the color will spread.

A spray bottle filled with clean water can give a different effect. With the scarf stretched above your work surface, lightly spray areas of your scarf with the water bottle. Don't spray too much water in one place, or the effect won't work as well. When you paint on the damp areas, the paint will have a softer bleeding effect. The water droplets may even make some of the paint spread more than others, resulting in a nice, textured effect.

Try it out on your practice papers to see how the colors move and change. The paints may act different-ly on the actual scarf than they do on the paper, but you can get a general idea of what the wet surface can do. And remember, if you accidentally get the scarf too wet, you can always let it dry before painting!

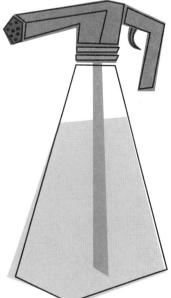

Is It Done Yet?

An important thing to remember when you're painting with these special fabric paints is that the scarf isn't really finished until it has dried and been *fixed*. Whenever the scarf is wet, you should be careful not to move it too much or allow one part of the scarf to touch another. If the colors are still wet and touch each other, they will blend together and may not look as nice. Once you've finished painting your scarf, you should let it dry on the stretcher sponges for at least twenty-four hours.

Even when the scarf is dry, the colors can still run or smear if they become wet before you've applied heat to the scarf to fix the colors. After the scarf has completely dried, put it in a clothes dryer by itself. Other clothes or scarves in the dryer could keep your decorated scarf from getting hot enough to make the paints permanent. Next, tumble dry the scarf on the high heat setting for ten to fifteen minutes.

Now your scarf should be ready to wear or give as a gift!

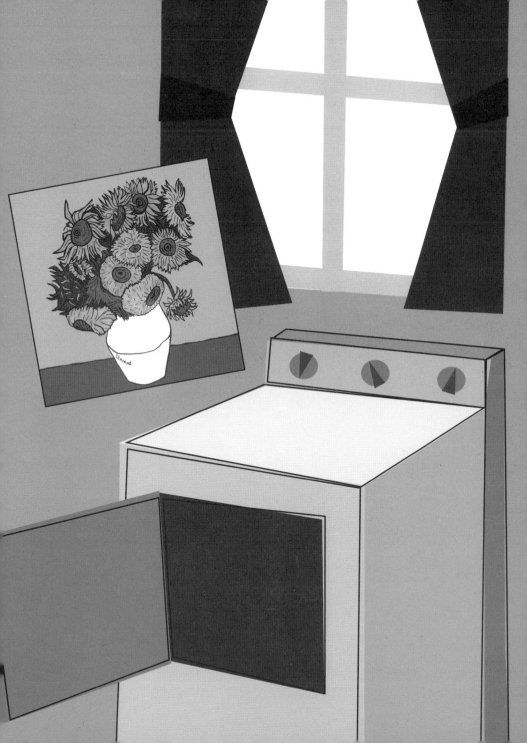

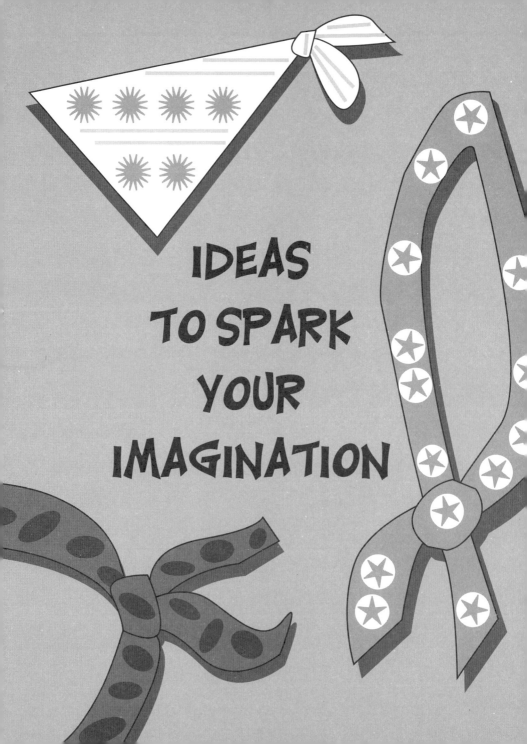

IDEAS
TO SPARK
YOUR
IMAGINATION

Painting a Masterpiece

The smaller, square scarf included in this kit already has an outline of a famous work of art by Vincent van Gogh printed on it. He painted *Fourteen Sunflowers in a Vase* in the summer of 1888 in Arles, France. Actually, van Gogh created *four* sunflower still-life paintings to decorate the room where his friend, another famous artist named Paul Gauguin, stayed when he came to Arles. In the end, he only liked two of them well enough to hang. One of the paintings was almost monochrome, or all one color. Van Gogh painted the flowers in different shades of yellow and orange, with a yellow background. The other painting had similar yellow and orange flowers, in front of a contrasting blue background. This version is the masterpiece that has been carefully redrawn and is ready for you to color with the paints—and your imagination. You can paint the image to look like van Gogh's, or you can ignore the lines and use one of the other painting methods in this book for a more abstract effect. You get to add whatever colors you want!

Van Gogh used strong brush strokes to express the emotion he felt when he looked at the large, blooming sunflowers. In his paintings, he didn't always "stay inside the lines," and you don't have to, either! If you've practiced with the colors, you know that they tend to travel through the paper or fabric. This is especially true if you get the surface wet first. If you want, you can make the paints spread and blend together like van Gogh did with his oil paints. With this method, the lines on the scarf aren't supposed to be boundaries for the colors, they're just details of the picture that will shine through the paint.

You can put more than one color in the same part of the picture. Just make sure that the colors blend well together if they are going to overlap. For instance, if red and yellow blend together you'll get bright orange. If red and green blend together, you'll get a muddy brown.

You might prefer to keep all the paint within the lines. In this technique, don't paint right up to the black lines as you add your colors to the image. Leave a little room for the color to move on its own and fill in the space between where you paint and the edge of the line. (It won't hurt your picture if there's some white left visible!)

Once you're done painting the picture, let the colors sit overnight and dry completely. Then fix the colors using the process described on page 24!

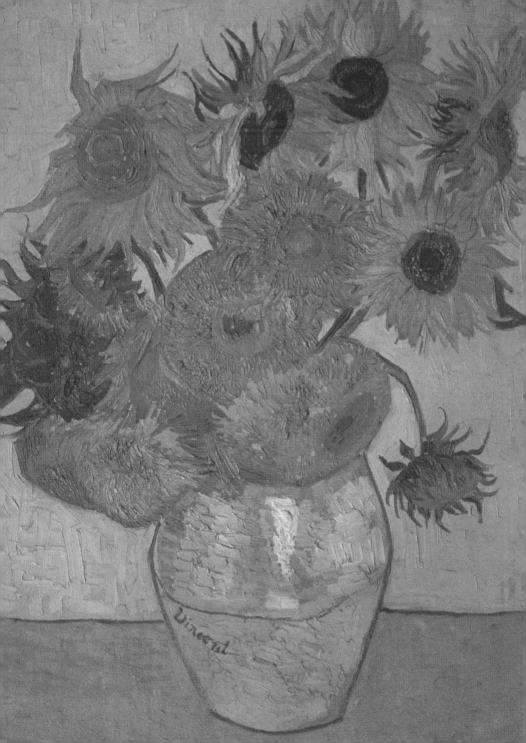

Drawing a Picture

After your brainstorming session, you may have chosen some pictures you want to draw on the blank scarf. Before you begin, practice painting your image on a practice sheet. Drawing with a crayon or marker is very different from painting the same thing with a paintbrush. Simple, basic shapes work better on the scarf material, since they won't mess up as easily if the paint spreads. Bigger pictures with fewer details also work very well on the

scarf surface, so keep that in mind as you're choosing your image and where it should go.

Once you're ready to start your painting, stretch the scarf on the stretcher sponges. It's very important not to get the scarf surface wet, so your paint won't bleed as much. Also, don't add any water to the brush. You

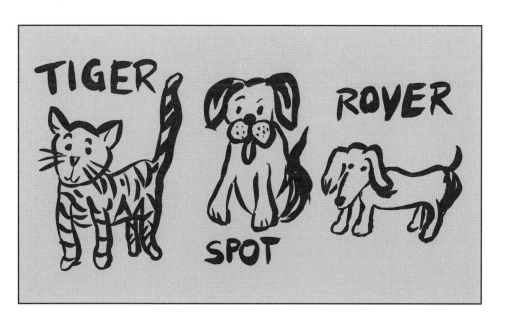

should dip the dry brush into your paint and then make a steady, broad stroke on the scarf. If the brush you are using is wet, gently pat it with a paper towel to take away the extra water. Remember that the image you draw won't look exactly like it did when you were using crayons or markers!

If you want to draw an outline or a picture over other colors, paint the colors first and then wait for them to dry completely. Then, use the technique described above. The most detailed part of your picture should be the last thing you paint so it doesn't get wet and smear. Don't forget that even mistakes can turn out to be beautiful!

Over the Rainbow

Many popular scarves have the colors of the rainbow, or at least some of them! You can use only the colors that came with the kit, or, if you want to get a little more involved, you can add violet (by mixing red and blue).

Once you have your scarf set up on the stretcher sponges, lightly wet the silk with water using a spray bottle. You'll want to paint fairly quickly, because the silk doesn't take long to dry out.

Starting at the lower left corner, paint large stripes of colors in this order:

RED

ORANGE

YELLOW

GREEN

BLUE

If you mixed orange and violet, the colors go in this order:

RED

ORANGE

YELLOW

GREEN

BLUE

VIOLET

As you paint, leave a gap between the stripes of colors. The color will spread through the fabric anyway. Or let them blend together for a real color wheel effect. Don't worry about the lines being perfect and straight!

When you're done, let the scarf sit overnight and dry completely. Fix the colors as described on page 24.

The White Stuff

For a fairly simple (but attractive!) blue and white scarf that looks like a summer sky, leave the fabric dry. Using the blue paint, draw outlines of several clouds on the scarf. Next, color in the area between the clouds, leaving the clouds themselves white. Make the brush really wet, and leave a little space between your brush strokes. You can also use the mixing tray to combine different amounts of water with the paint to create some color variations in the blue sky. Think about adding other things to the sky, like the sun, a colorful kite, or a butterfly or bird.

You could also use this technique of leaving some white on the scarf with other designs. You might want to leave smaller areas of white in the shape of stars to create a clear night sky. Or, you could use white space to create a snow scene, with snowmen or a snow-capped mountain. White space could also be used as a border, or to separate pictures in different areas of the scarf. Use your imagination to make the most of the unpainted scarf!

A Pinch of Salt

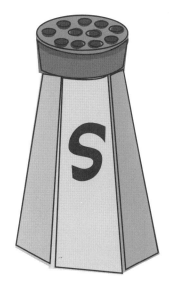

For this project, you'll need to get some rock salt. You can use it to make natural patterns in your painting! Kosher salt or table salt will also work, but the pattern won't be as dramatic.

Paint the entire scarf with one or more colors. Once you have finished painting, very lightly spray the scarf with water. (Not too much!)

Next, take the rock salt and scatter it across the scarf. Let it sit on the scarf until the paint has dried. When you're sure the paint is dry, carefully pour the salt off the silk into the trash. Every spot that had salt will have a lighter-colored pattern underneath it.

Instead of just sprinkling the salt across the whole scarf, you can also make patterns with it. Try laying stripes of salt diagonally across the scarf or making a starburst pattern!

Circle, Circle, Dot, Dot

If you go wild for polka dots, choose two colors that blend well together, a light one and a dark one. Experiment with your choices on the template paper until you get two that you like together.

Once your scarf is set up on the stretcher sponges, completely paint the scarf with the lighter color. Then, while the scarf is still wet, dip the brush in the darker color and gently put spots of color on the scarf. The paint will travel and blend with the lighter color. You can either make the dots look random in size or location, or you can make a pattern out of them.

Let the paint dry. To make some lighter dots, take a clean brush and wet it with water. Then, dab the brush on the scarf. The water will spread through the paint and make new spots. You can also put the water dots into the center of the dark colored dots for another shade of the same color. When you've got enough dots to make you happy, let the paint dry overnight and then fix the colors.

You can use the same technique with other shapes. Repeat the pattern in the same size or different sizes all over the scarf. Just be careful to choose a shape that is easy to draw and won't get messed up if the paint spreads out a bit.

Scarf Stripes

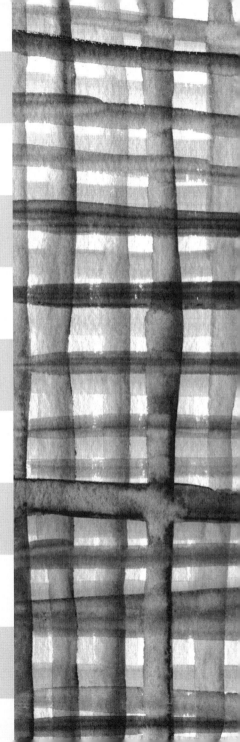

For a plaid or checkered effect, pick or mix one main color for your scarf and completely paint the scarf with it. Before the paint dries, take a clean brush dipped in plain water and use it to draw lines on the scarf. It should leave a lighter-colored stripe on the scarf. (Don't worry about getting the lines perfect—that's part of the handmade look!) Rinse the brush a little each time you dip it into the water to keep it clean. After the stripes have been put on, you could also put little water-dabs in the squares created by the grid, or add small dots in another color!

When you finish your stripes, let the paint dry overnight and then fix the colors.

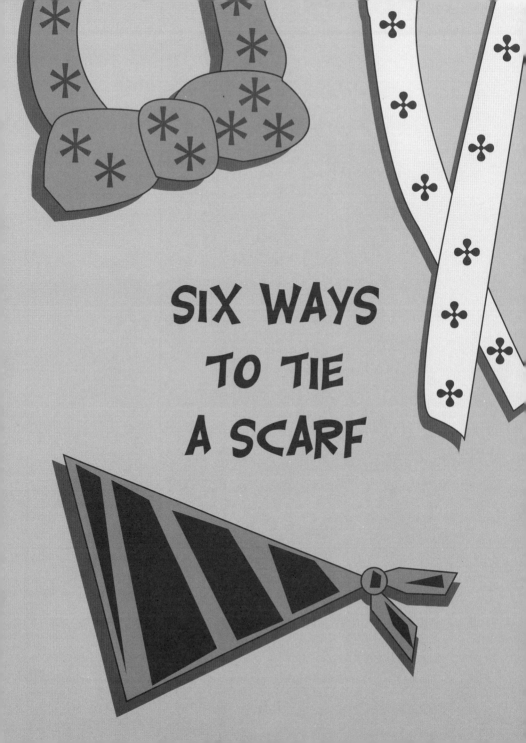

SIX WAYS TO TIE A SCARF

Now that you've finished creating your artistic scarves, it's time for them to be worn. (Assuming the paint is completely dry, of course!) There are many ways to wear and tie a scarf.

Scarves can be worn on the head, around the neck, or draped over the shoulders. A long scarf can even be tied around the waist and used as a belt or sash. Some people use their scarves as decoration for a wall or chair.

Whether you are making scarves for yourself or to give as a gift you might want to learn some different ways to tie a scarf. Some methods work best with the long, rectangular scarf and others work better for the smaller square one. A few will work with either shape of scarf. All of them will show off your special creations!

The Loop is as simple as it comes and works well with the rectangular scarf.

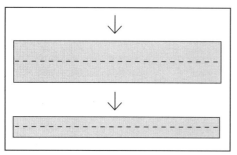

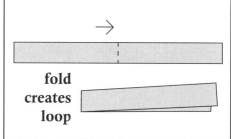

fold
creates
loop

1. Fold the short side of your scarf in half twice so it is about three inches wide.

2. Fold the long side in half.

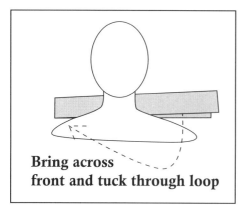

Bring across
front and tuck through loop

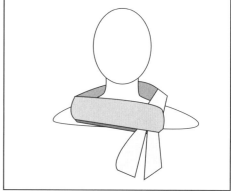

3. Drape the folded scarf across the back of your neck.

4. Pull the two loose ends of the scarf through the loop made by the fold.

The Basic Head Wrap is perfect for either scarf shape. Who needs

a hat? Use your own scarf instead!

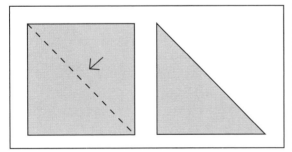

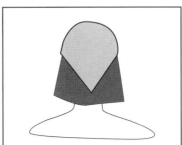

1. Fold the square scarf into a triangle. (Or, for the rectangular scarf, don't fold it at all.)

2. Lay the scarf across your head so the point of the triangle rests on the back of your neck (or so the long ends of the rectangular scarf are over your ears).

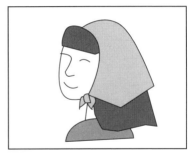

3. Tie the corners of the triangle across the back of your head under your hair, just above the neck. Or, tie the long ends of the rectangular scarf under your chin. You could also tie the square scarf over your hair and tuck the point of the triangle under the knot.

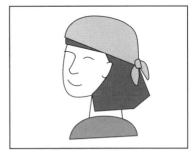

The Tie uses the rectangular scarf and wraps around the neck like a loose necktie.

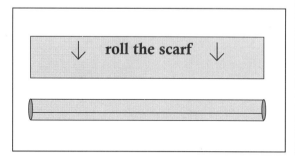

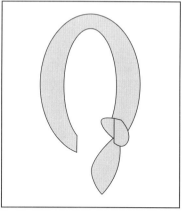

1. Roll the scarf into a long strip about two inches wide.

2. Tie a knot in one end about ten inches from the tip.

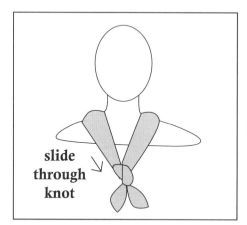

slide through knot

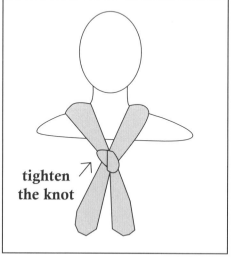

tighten the knot

3. Loop the other end around your neck, with the middle of the scarf laying across the back of your neck.

4. Pull the other end through the knot and tighten slightly.

The Basic Bandana Neckerchief will really show off your

painting on the square scarf!

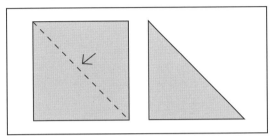

1. Fold the scarf in half to make a triangle.

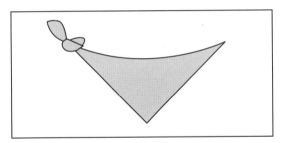

2. Tie a simple knot in one corner of the long side of the triangle, about one inch from the end.

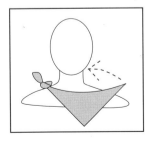

3. Bring the end with the knot in front of your neck.

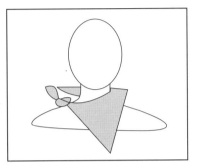

4. Pass the corner without the knot behind your neck. Thread the corner through the knot, pulling it through to match the other corner.

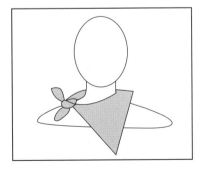

5. Place the knot on one side of your neck, and drape the scarf just in front of your shoulder.

The Bow Not Knot uses the larger scarf to make what *looks* like a

bow, but is easier to tie!

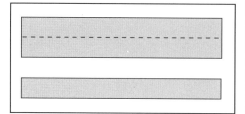

1. Fold the scarf in half lengthwise.

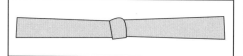

2. Tie a large, loose knot in the center of the scarf.

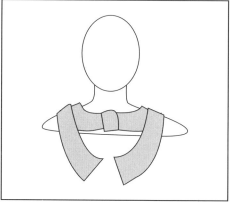

4. Bring the ends back around your neck to the front.

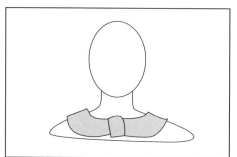

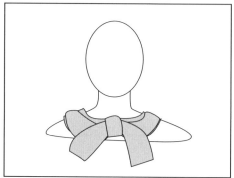

3. Wrap the ends around the back of your neck, with the knot centered under your chin.

5. Pass the ends through the knot. Pull them through and fluff them a bit. Tighten the knot.

The Rolled Neckerchief is a quick and simple knot that has a

European flair to it. It uses the square scarf.

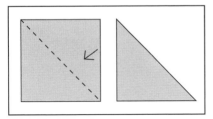 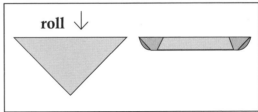

1. Fold the scarf in half to make a triangle and roll the scarf into a strip about one inch wide.

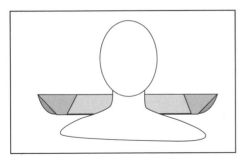 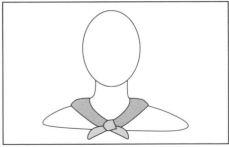

2. Pull the scarf across the back of your neck and tie the ends in a simple knot in the front.

3. Fluff out the ends of the knot, and position slightly off to one side of your neck.

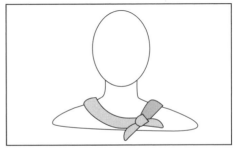

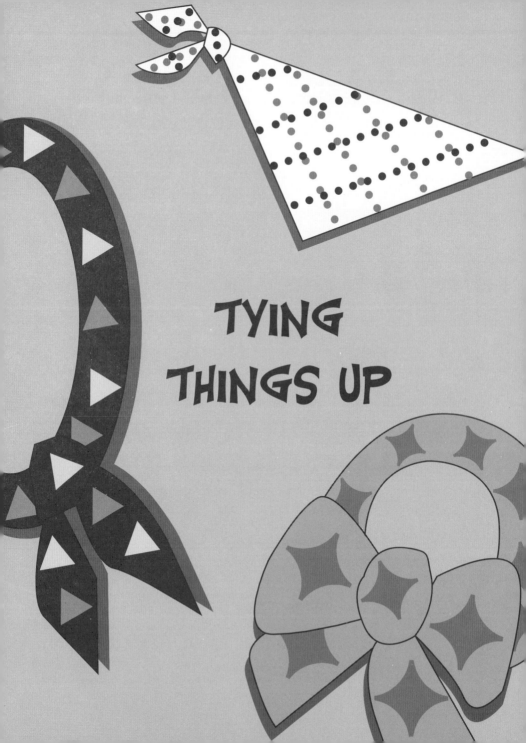

TYING
THINGS UP

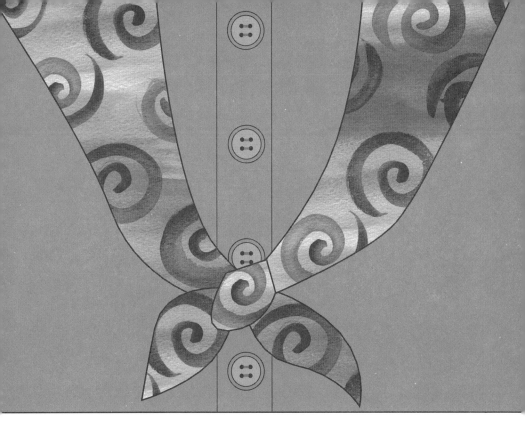

ow that you've created your two original scarves, you have joined a long tradition that reaches back thousands of years. You can use crayons, colored pencils, or markers to decorate the gift box included in this kit. Then, carefully fold the scarf or scarves into the box and deliver it with pride. Your one-of-a-kind artwork will stand out in the crowd of hum-drum everyday neckwear, and the person you give it to will wear it with pride. Congratulations!

ABOUT THE AUTHOR

Conn McQuinn has spent 24 years working

in education, and has written more

than a dozen children's books. He also wrote

the books for *The Ultimate Tie Kit* and *Build Your*

Own FM Radio (both published by Running Press).

He lives in Burien, Washington with his wife,

two children, and a variety of animals.